Knee osteoarthritis

All you need to know

Dr. Sheila Harrison

Disclaimer

This content serves to provide general information about the disease and aims to empower you to seek prompt medical assistance if necessary to prevent complications. It's essential to stress that this information is not a substitute for consulting a qualified physician. The field of medical science is continually evolving, and due to the dynamic nature of medical knowledge, we recommend seeking expert advice if you encounter any inconsistencies or intend to take action based on the information in this content. Never disregard professional medical guidance or delay treatment based on something you've read online, including this material, or from any other online source. Always remember that the internet cannot cure you; rather, healing comes through the guidance of medical professionals and the providence of God.

Table of contents

Introduction

Osteoarthritis, commonly referred to as OA, stands as the most prevalent form of arthritis that affects a vast number of individuals across the globe. This condition is characterized by the progressive degeneration of joint cartilage and the underlying bone. While osteoarthritis can manifest in various joints in the body, it frequently targets the knee joints, leading to an increased risk of fractures in the femur, tibia, or patella.

Normal Knee

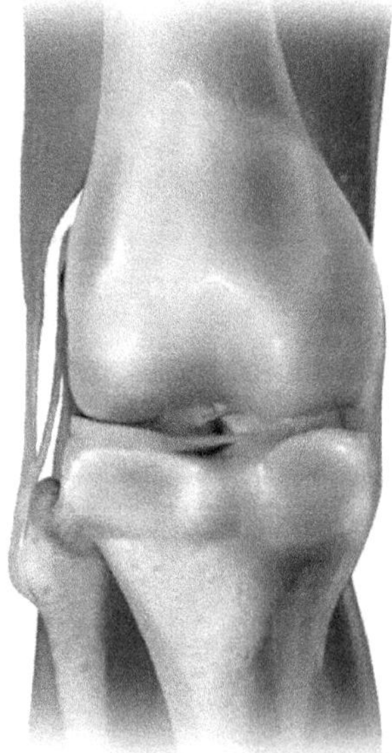

Osteoarthritis

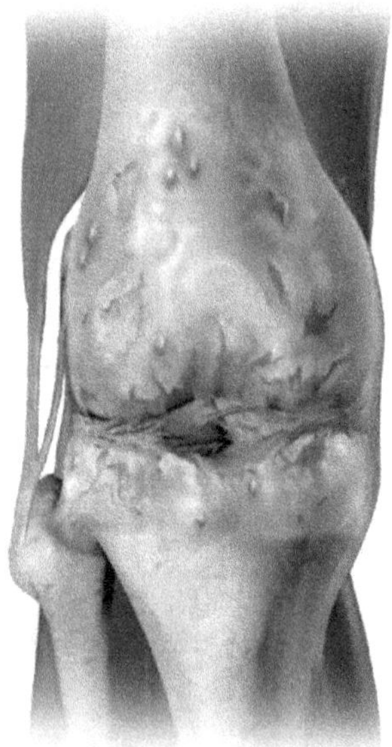

Section 1

OVERVIEW (Knee Osteoarthritis)

One striking aspect of knee osteoarthritis is that it does not discriminate based on age. This condition can affect individuals of any age, making it a concern across the lifespan. However, the risk of developing knee osteoarthritis significantly escalates after the age of forty-five. As individuals grow older, the wear and tear on their bodies accumulate, impacting the health of their knee joints.

Knee osteoarthritis is a multifaceted condition with a range of factors contributing to its development. Infection is one potential cause; however, it is less common than other influences. In cases where an infection takes hold within the knee joint, it can result in inflammation, damage to cartilage, and changes to joint tissues that can lead to osteoarthritis.

Another major contributor to the development and progression of knee osteoarthritis is obesity.

Excess body weight places significant stress on the knee joints, accelerating the wear and tear process. The cartilage that cushions the ends of bones becomes more vulnerable to damage as it struggles to bear the additional load. Consequently, obesity significantly amplifies the risk of knee osteoarthritis.

Hormonal changes and genetic predispositions are known to play roles in the development of knee osteoarthritis. These factors can make certain individuals more vulnerable to the condition. While there is ongoing research to better understand the influence of hormones and genetics on osteoarthritis, it is apparent that they contribute to the complexity of this multifactorial disease.

Notably, knee osteoarthritis reveals a gender-related discrepancy. Women are more susceptible to developing osteoarthritis in the knee joints compared to men. This discrepancy is influenced by a combination of factors, including hormonal variations, differences in joint alignment, and genetic predispositions.

The Global Scale of Knee Osteoarthritis

A study published in the respected Lancet journal in 2020 provided a stark revelation regarding the prevalence of knee osteoarthritis. The research estimated that a staggering 654.1 million individuals aged forty or older were living with knee osteoarthritis across the world. These numbers underscore the enormous impact of this condition on people's lives and the significant healthcare burden it places on society.

Knee Osteoarthritis in the United States

Knee osteoarthritis is a major health concern in the United States, particularly among older adults and individuals with specific risk factors. The prevalence of knee osteoarthritis in people over the age of forty varies from 16% to 23%, with higher rates observed in older age groups. The economic burden of knee osteoarthritis is substantial, encompassing healthcare costs associated with diagnosis, treatment, and management.

Individuals who suffer from knee osteoarthritis face numerous challenges. Fractures, chronic pain, and associated complications compromise their quality of life, mobility, and independence. This not only affects individuals but also has a significant societal impact.

The Need for Long-Term Care

One common outcome of knee osteoarthritis is the requirement for long-term home care due to the chronic discomfort it causes. This added strain on healthcare systems, families, and individuals is a considerable concern.

To sum up, knee osteoarthritis is a complicated ailment with a variety of risk factors that add to its high incidence and significant financial burden on both individuals and society. The well-being of individuals with knee osteoarthritis and the healthcare systems that serve them depends on efforts to better understand, prevent, and manage the condition.

Section 2

Symptoms of knee osteoarthritis

Some of the prevalent symptoms of knee osteoarthritis include the following:

- **Pain:** The most typical sign of osteoarthritis in the knee joint is persistent pain. The pain can be either subtle or acute, and it can get worse when you walk, climb stairs, or remain still for a long time. Moreover, pain may worsen during periods of inactivity.

- **Stiffness:** One prevalent sign of knee osteoarthritis is stiffness in the knee joint, especially after extended periods of rest or inactivity. Moving or bending the knee may be difficult if it feels stiff and unnatural..

- **Swelling:** One sign of osteoarthritis in the knee is swelling or inflammation in the joint. The joint may feel heated to the touch, have a noticeable swollen appearance, and feel tight.

- **Reduced Mobility:** Another symptom of knee osteoarthritis is the decrease in the knee joint's range of motion. It may become difficult to fully straighten or bend the knee, limiting flexibility and mobility.

- **Crepitus:** Crepitus is one of the most prevalent signs of osteoarthritis in the knee. When a person moves their knee joint, they may feel or hear a crackling or grating sound. This noise is the result of the cartilage inside the joint wearing down or becoming abrasive.

- **Weakness:** Muscle weakness in the knee joint is a possible symptom of osteoarthritis in some people. This weakness may be a factor in instability as well as balance and walking issues.

- **Functional Limitations:** As knee osteoarthritis worsens, people may find it more difficult to carry out regular tasks including walking, climbing stairs, and rising from a seated position. The overall quality of life may be considerably impacted by these functional restrictions.

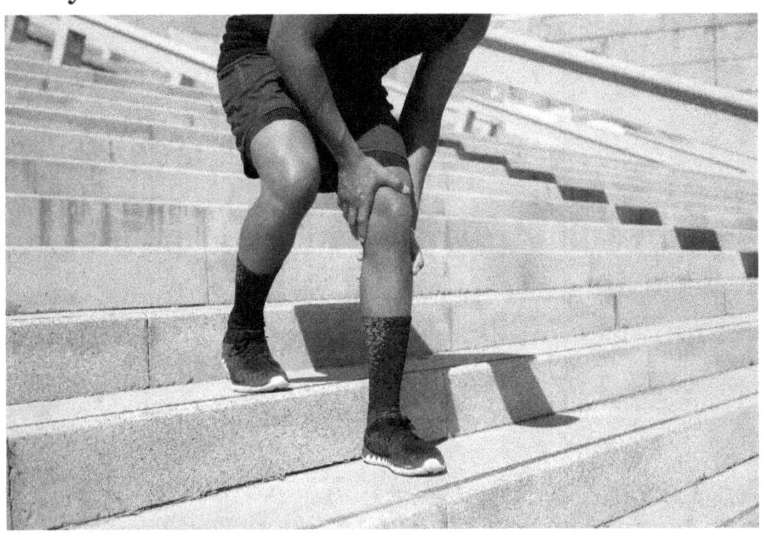

Section 3

Causes of knee osteoarthritis

The causes of knee osteoarthritis can be multifactorial, involving a combination of genetic, biomechanical, and lifestyle factors. Here are some common causes:

- **Chronic injury and joint stress:** People who spend a lot of time on their feet, and do heavy lifting while standing, squatting, or crawling frequently may have 'mini-traumas' in their knee joints. This can cause knee osteoarthritis.

- **Lack of physical activity:** While too much strain on the knee joint can lead to arthritis, so can a lack of it. To promote cartilage health and repair, the knee joint cartilage must be subjected to weight-bearing stress. Prolonged lack of physical activity can also cause knee osteoarthritis.

- **Muscle tone issues:** When the hamstring, quadriceps, and calf muscles are weak, the knee cartilage and underlying bone endure greater stress. Knee osteoarthritis can develop as a result of this.

- **Biochemical changes:** Research has identified certain biochemical abnormalities in knee joints that osteoarthritis causes.

- **Joint Misalignment:** Abnormal alignment of the knee joint, such as bowlegs or knock knees, can place uneven stress on the joint surfaces, leading to increased wear and tear.

Section 4

Risk factors associated with knee osteoarthritis

- **Age:** With increasing age, the cartilage undergoes more wear and tear, and its ability to mend decreases.

- **Weight:** Strain can occur on a joint due to an increase in weight, particularly on the knees. Every pound acquired may add 3 to 4 pounds of additional weight to the knees.

- **Heredity:** This includes genetic changes that may increase a person's risk of developing osteoarthritis.

- **Gender:** Osteoarthritis of the knee affects more women than men.

Repetitive stress injuries (RSIs)

These injuries occur when repeated stress occurs on a joint. This usually depends on a person's occupation. People who work in jobs that require a lot of physical activity that strains the joints are more prone to developing osteoarthritis.

- **Athletes:** Athletes who participate in soccer, tennis, or long-distance running may be more likely to develop osteoarthritis of the knee.

- **Other diseases:** Osteoarthritis is more common in people who have rheumatoid arthritis. This type of osteoarthritis occurs in those with another joint disease, called secondary arthritis.

- **Metabolic issues:** Osteoarthritis is more common in those with metabolic problems, such as iron overload or excess growth hormone.

Section 5

Diagnosis process of knee osteoarthritis?

Knee osteoarthritis is typically diagnosed through clinical evaluation, medical history assessment, and diagnostic imaging. The following are the common methods for the diagnosis of knee osteoarthritis:

Medical history

The healthcare provider will discuss your symptoms, their duration, and any previous injuries or medical conditions that may be contributing to your knee pain.

Physical examination

A physical examination by your doctor will be the first step in the diagnosis of knee osteoarthritis. The healthcare provider will perform a physical examination of your knee joint, assessing its range of motion, stability, and signs of inflammation. They may also look for joint swelling, tenderness, and the presence of crepitus (a crackling sound) during movement.

Imaging studies

Various imaging techniques may be used to evaluate the knee joint and confirm the diagnosis of osteoarthritis. These may include:

- **X-rays:** Knee osteoarthritis X-ray images provide detailed structures of the bones and can reveal joint space narrowing, bone spurs, and other characteristic changes associated with osteoarthritis. X-rays show bone and cartilage deterioration as well as the existence of bone spurs. This may aid in the diagnosis of knee osteoarthritis. When X-rays do not reveal a clear cause for joint discomfort or when the X-rays indicate that other types of joint tissue may be injured, MRI scans may be ordered.

- **Magnetic Resonance Imaging (MRI):** MRI scans use powerful magnets and radio waves to produce detailed images of the knee joint, including the cartilage, ligaments, and surrounding soft tissues. This can help assess the extent of cartilage damage and identify other possible causes of knee pain.

- **Ultrasound:** Ultrasound imaging can be used to visualize soft tissues, such as the synovium and ligaments, and may help identify inflammation or fluid accumulation within the joint.

- **Laboratory Tests:** While there are no specific blood tests for the diagnosis of knee osteoarthritis, blood tests may be ordered to rule out other conditions that can mimic osteoarthritis, such as rheumatoid arthritis.

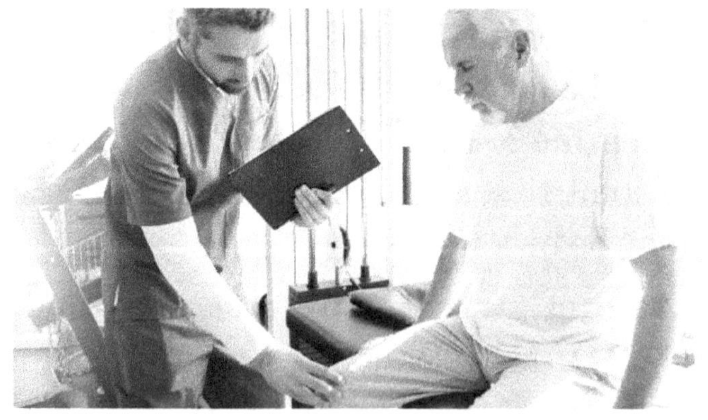

Section 6

Complications associated with knee osteoarthritis

Knee osteoarthritis is a condition that brings about a range of complications, significantly impacting the lives of those affected. Here, we will delve into some of the key complications associated with knee osteoarthritis.

- **Stiffness and Pain:** One of the primary complications of knee osteoarthritis is the persistent stiffness and pain that it inflicts on individuals. As the condition progresses, the joints in the knee become less flexible and more rigid, leading to stiffness. This stiffness can be particularly pronounced in the morning or after prolonged periods of inactivity. Pain is another hallmark of knee osteoarthritis. The pain is often localized to the affected knee joint and can range from mild discomfort to severe agony. It may be constant or occur during certain activities, such as walking or standing. This chronic pain and stiffness have a profound impact on a person's daily life, affecting their ability to perform routine tasks and enjoy regular activities.

- **Physical and Mobility Challenges:** Knee osteoarthritis has a cascading effect on an individual's physical abilities and mobility. As the condition worsens, it leads to physical limitations that make everyday movements and tasks increasingly challenging. Individuals with knee osteoarthritis frequently find it difficult to engage in activities that were once routine, such as walking, climbing stairs, or even standing for extended periods. The pain and stiffness associated with knee osteoarthritis hinder the free movement of the joint, making bending and flexing the knee joint arduous.

- **Impact on Daily Activities:** The complications of knee osteoarthritis extend beyond the physical realm and affect one's ability to carry out daily activities. Something as fundamental as walking may become a painful and laborious task. The pain and discomfort experienced during weight-bearing activities can lead to significant limitations, impacting an individual's independence. Tasks like going to the grocery store, taking a stroll in the park, or visiting friends and family become increasingly challenging.

- **Impaired Quality of Life:** Knee osteoarthritis not only affects physical well-being but also significantly impairs one's quality of life. The discomfort, pain, and reduced mobility often lead to frustration and a diminished sense of well-being. The limitations that knee osteoarthritis imposes can also have emotional and psychological consequences, causing feelings of sadness, anxiety, or even depression.

- **Reduced Participation in Activities:** As knee osteoarthritis progresses and complications intensify, individuals may begin to withdraw from various activities they once enjoyed. They may avoid engaging in physical and social activities that involve movement due to the fear of pain or further joint damage. Consequently, their social lives may be impacted as they participate less in group activities or gatherings.

- **Challenges in Self-Care:** The daily activities of self-care, such as bathing, dressing, and grooming, can also become challenging for individuals with knee osteoarthritis. Simple tasks like bending down to tie shoelaces or getting in and out of the shower can become arduous. These challenges in self-care can erode an individual's sense of independence.

As a whole, people with knee osteoarthritis experience a variety of life difficulties. A person's quality of life might be negatively impacted, their daily routines can be disturbed, and they may experience emotional and social difficulties as a result of pain, stiffness, and limitations in their physical mobility and activity. Having an understanding of these issues is essential to creating efficient strategies to manage knee osteoarthritis and improve the well-being of those living with this condition.

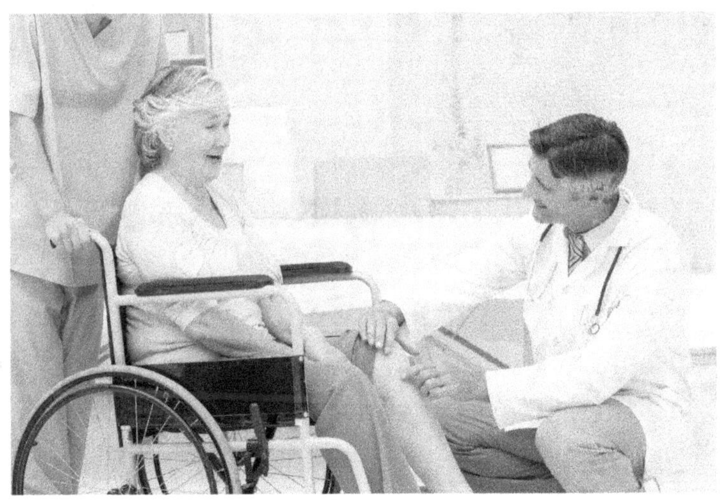

Section 7

Treatment of knee osteoarthritis

The treatment of knee osteoarthritis aims to alleviate pain, improve joint function, and enhance the individual's overall quality of life. The treatment approach may involve a combination of non-pharmacological interventions, medications, and, in severe cases, surgical options. Here are some common treatment strategies for knee osteoarthritis:

Non-Pharmacological Interventions:

- **Weight management:** Maintaining a healthy weight or losing excess weight can reduce stress on the knee joint.

- **Exercise and physical therapy:** Strengthening exercises, low-impact aerobic activities, and flexibility exercises can help improve joint stability, and mobility, and reduce pain.

- **Assistive devices:** The use of assistive devices like braces, orthotics, or walking aids can provide support and reduce pressure on the knee joint.

- **Hot and cold therapy:** Applying heat or cold packs to the knee can help alleviate pain and inflammation.

Pharmacological Interventions:

- **Analgesics:** Over-the-counter pain relievers like acetaminophen or nonsteroidal anti-inflammatory drugs (NSAIDs) can help manage pain and reduce inflammation.

- **Topical Medications:** Creams, gels, or patches containing NSAIDs or capsaicin can be applied directly to the knee joint for localized pain relief.

- **Intra-Articular Injections:** Corticosteroids or hyaluronic acid injections can relieve temporary pain and reduce inflammation in the knee joint.

Surgical Interventions:

- **Arthroscopy:** Minimally invasive surgery to repair or remove damaged tissue within the knee joint.

- **Osteotomy:** A surgical procedure that involves reshaping or realigning the bones to relieve pressure on the damaged area.

- **Total Knee Replacement:** In severe cases, the damaged knee joint may be replaced with an artificial joint made of metal and plastic components. You must consult the doctor as they will suggest to you when to undergo knee replacement surgery.

Complementary and Alternative Therapies:

- **Acupuncture:** The insertion of thin needles into specific points on the body to help reduce pain and improve symptoms.

- **Herbal Supplements:** Some herbal supplements, such as glucosamine and chondroitin sulfate, are believed to provide symptom relief, although scientific evidence is mixed.

The choice of treatment depends on various factors, including the severity of symptoms, individual preferences, and the healthcare provider's recommendations.

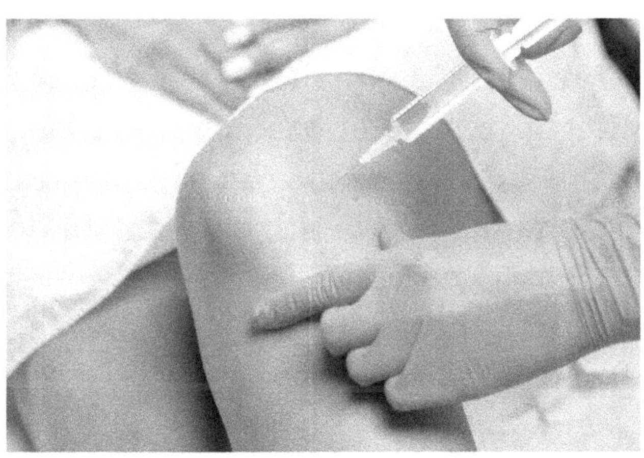

Section 8

Prevention of knee osteoarthritis

While it may not be possible to prevent knee osteoarthritis entirely, certain lifestyle modifications and strategies can help reduce the risk or delay the onset of the condition.

The following measures will help in the general health of the knees and may prevent the development and progression of knee osteoarthritis:

- **Maintain a healthy weight:** Excess weight puts additional stress on the knee joints, increasing the risk of osteoarthritis. Maintaining a healthy weight or losing weight if necessary can help reduce the load on the joints and may prevent you from knee osteoarthritis.

- **Exercise regularly:** Exercise helps strengthen the muscles around the knee joint, improves joint stability, and supports overall joint health. Regular exercise may prevent you from knee osteoarthritis. Engage in regular exercise that includes a combination of cardiovascular activities, strength training, and flexibility exercises.

- **Protect your joints:** When participating in sports or physical activities, use appropriate protective equipment, such as knee pads, to minimize the risk of knee injuries that can lead to osteoarthritis.

- **Practice good posture and body mechanics:** Maintain proper posture and body mechanics during activities such as sitting, standing, lifting, and bending to minimize excessive stress on the knee joints.

- **Avoid repetitive knee stress:** Limit activities that involve repetitive stress on the knees, such as kneeling, squatting, or prolonged periods of standing, especially on hard surfaces. This may aid in the prevention of knee osteoarthritis.

- **Use joint-supporting footwear:** Wear comfortable and supportive shoes that provide cushioning and shock absorption to reduce the impact on the knee joints.

- **Warm up and cool down:** Before engaging in physical activities, warm up your muscles and joints with gentle exercises and stretching. Afterwards, cool down and stretch to help maintain flexibility and prevent muscle tightness.

- **Maintain a healthy lifestyle:** Adopt a healthy lifestyle that includes a balanced diet rich in nutrients, adequate hydration, and avoiding smoking, as smoking has been associated with an increased risk of osteoarthritis.

Section 9

FAQ on Knee Osteoarthritis

Are diabetes and knee osteoarthritis related?

Diabetes and knee osteoarthritis share risk factors like obesity and inflammation. They can indirectly affect each other due to limited physical activity caused by osteoarthritis and potential medication interactions. Managing both conditions requires close medical supervision and lifestyle adjustments.

Can knee osteoarthritis affect kidney diseases?

Knee osteoarthritis and kidney diseases primarily affect different parts of the body. But they may indirectly influence each other due to shared risk factors, medications, inflammation, and reduced physical activity.

Can knee osteoarthritis cause heart problems?

No, knee osteoarthritis does not directly cause heart problems. It is a degenerative joint disease affecting the cartilage and bones, not the heart. However, some risk factors associated with osteoarthritis, such as obesity and inactivity, may contribute to developing heart issues over time.

Can knee osteoarthritis cause liver problems?

Knee osteoarthritis is primarily a joint-related condition and does not directly cause liver problems. However, certain medications used to manage knee osteoarthritis, such as acetaminophen (paracetamol) and nonsteroidal anti-inflammatory drugs (NSAIDs), can potentially affect the liver when used excessively or inappropriately. Prolonged or high-dose use of these medications can contribute to liver damage.

Does high cholesterol cause knee osteoarthritis?

There is no direct evidence to suggest that high cholesterol causes knee osteoarthritis. Osteoarthritis primarily results from wear and tear on the joints over time, genetic factors, and other risk factors such as age, obesity, and joint injuries. However, high cholesterol levels and related conditions like obesity can contribute to other health issues that may indirectly affect joint health and exacerbate osteoarthritis.

Why is knee osteoarthritis a sign of weak bones?

Knee osteoarthritis is not a direct sign of weak bones. It is a degenerative joint disease that primarily affects the cartilage in the joints, not the bones themselves. However, underlying bone health can play a role in the development and progression of osteoarthritis. Factors such as reduced bone density or osteoporosis can weaken the support for joints, potentially increasing the risk of joint damage and worsening osteoarthritis symptoms. So, while osteoarthritis is not a sign of weak bones per se, the overall health of the bones can impact the condition's severity and progression.